WEIGHT
NO MORE

ANNE HUNT

Edited by Eric Mein, M.D.

A Note to the Reader

The information in this book is not presented as prescription for the treatment of disease. Application of the medical information found in the Edgar Cayce readings and interpreted herein should be undertaken only under the supervision of a physician.

Other Books in This Series

SAVING YOUR SKIN: Secrets of Healthy Skin and Hair
WINNING THE COLD WAR: Preventing and Curing the Common Cold and Flu

Copyright © 1990
by the
Edgar Cayce Foundation
All rights reserved.

ISBN 87604-260-4

2nd Printing, June 1991

Printed in the U.S.A.

Table of Contents

Preface by Mark Thurston, Ph.D.   V

Introduction by Eric Mein, M.D.   IX

Chapter One	Who Needs to Diet?	1
Chapter Two	The Body, Mind, and Spirit Diet	6
Chapter Three	How to Get Started	12
Chapter Four	Mental Muscle	24
Chapter Five	Building a Healthier Body	35
Chapter Six	Can-Do Diet and Exercise Tips	44
Chapter Seven	The Four-Week Therapy Program	58
Conclusion		66
Appendix A	Who Was Edgar Cayce?	68
Appendix B	How the A.R.E. Can Help You	70
Appendix C	How to Obtain a Pre-sleep Tape for Weight Loss	72
Appendix D	Directions for Self-Administered Therapies	73

Acknowledgments

Much of the information presented in this book is based on materials developed by Mark Thurston, Lynn Sparrow, and Henry Reed for the A.R.E. Conference "Secrets of Weight Control." Douglas Richards also played a role in synthesizing this material in A.R.E.'s Home Study Research Project also entitled "Secrets of Weight Control."

PREFACE

It's no secret that our society is in the midst of a health care crisis. The problem is partly economic, as we struggle to find ways to pay for the high level of care made possible by medical technology. It's also a research crisis, as scientists look for cures to new diseases such as AIDS. Those are the sorts of problems that make the headlines. Those are the challenges that are clearly evident.

But our health care crisis has more subtle features, too—aspects that are easy to miss but just as important. For example, how much guarantee can doctors give us for our health? How much responsibility are we willing to accept *for ourselves?* Are there some ailments for which *self-care* is not only more economical but also more likely to produce the results we want?

Another elusive feature of our society's health care crisis is in our attitude toward health and healing itself. Recent decades have seen an explosion of alternative health services, many of them claiming to follow a more natural or a more holistic approach. The success of some of these new methods makes us wonder about the validity of the familiar medical model. Is the body really more or less a machine that gets fixed like a balky appliance or a malfunctioning vehicle? Or is the human being a rich, complex mixture of body, mind, and spirit where problems at one level must be addressed at all three?

Working in the first four-and-a-half decades of the twentieth century, Edgar Cayce was a tremendous resource that we can now draw upon to meet the modern crisis in health care. His approach and methods for health maintenance and healing feature self-care that is often, yet not always, in conjunction with a physician's guidance. He was truly a pioneer of the contemporary holistic health movement and ahead of his times in pointing out the attitudinal, emotional, and spiritual components of disease.

Although best known as a "psychic" (or "the sleeping prophet," referring to his occasional predictions about world conditions), Cayce might be better labeled as a "clairvoyant diagnostician" or an "intuitive physician." The point with these descriptive terms is to emphasize first that Cayce's work was principally diagnostic and prescriptive. He was not a healer nor did he have office hours to see patients the way a doctor would. The cases that he took, the people who came to him for help were almost invariably those who had unsuccessfully tried the traditional medical approaches of their day and came to Cayce as a last resort, asking "What's *really* wrong with me? What treatments—no matter how unusual—will bring relief and healing?"

But as the descriptive labels for Cayce also

emphasize, his method of meeting those requests was intuitive. He had no formal medical school training. Yet he was apparently able to alter his consciousness in such a way that he could see clairvoyantly the real origins of afflictions (physical, mental, and spiritual). What's more, he could then prescribe natural and holistic treatment procedures—sometimes requiring the involvement of a physician or other health care professional, but often needing only a self-care regimen.

The material came through as lengthy discourses (called "readings"), which were stenographically recorded and then transcribed. Most of the information was given for specific individuals and their afflictions, but on occasion there were readings given on particular health topics which contained universally applicable information.

This book is one of a series of volumes in which common ailments and health difficulties are directed. Each topic addresses information given by Cayce which is principally focused upon self-care. The author, Anne Hunt, has carefully researched those readings on the respective health concern, focusing on the treatment procedures that were suggested to many different people as well as those recommendations that were clearly indicated for general use. Her research compilation and writing go a long way toward making these helpful methods accessible to us all. You'll find all the books in this series highly readable and very practical.

Anne's collaborator is Dr. Eric Mein, who served as medical editor. Sometimes Cayce's language requires the insight of a trained physician to translate concepts into modern terminology. Often there are new findings in medical research that shed light on one of Cayce's ideas. Eric has skillfully added that dimension to the creation of this book.

This particular volume in the series focuses on weight control. Does the world need yet another program for how to lose weight? Is the Cayce regimen to be just another fad? Yes and no. Yes, there *is* room for another answer to the weight-control question if we realize how few (if any) of the current offerings deal with the issue from a spiritual viewpoint. No, the Cayce approach isn't likely to become a fad. It has the appeal of being simple and straightforward, but it requires work on all three levels: body, mind, and spirit. This is no quick fix. It's a life-style alteration that takes time but promises the reward of lasting change in how you feel about your body and how it looks. The Cayce readings don't claim to have *the* answer to this health dilemma, but they do offer a highly practical, self-care approach to overall prevention as well as treatment.

Mark Thurston, Ph.D.
Association for Research and Enlightenment, Inc.

INTRODUCTION

In our society the issues surrounding body weight are complex. Each year, millions of Americans armed with misinformation launch themselves on another fad diet, often at great expense to themselves. In their frenzy to be thin, they are often willing to try bizarre gimmicks and believe outlandish promises. Much of the information that is routinely told to us concerning the losing or gaining of fat is either misleading or meaningless. The fact that one diet program after another appears on the best-seller list is proof that none has the ultimate answer. Despite this, more than ten billion dollars a year is spent on diet pills, diet books, weight-reduction centers, special diet foods and beverages, and other accessories in the bid for slenderness.

Yet this issue is a very real concern. An estimated 80 million Americans are overweight, and 20 million American adults are "on a diet" at any given time. Clearly, losing weight is not as simple as being strong-willed and going on a strict diet. Even when people succeed in the short haul, four out of five who have successfully lost weight through dieting will eventually regain it, often exceeding their previous high-weight mark.

While the reducing diet is not an effective means of weight control, it does, however, represent a ritual of self-improvement and self-purification which is admirable. Successful, permanent weight loss is more likely to occur given the "right motive." Dietary choices made for reasons of health and belief stand a better chance of changing one's deeply ingrained habits.

The holistic approach to weight control that you'll find within these pages focuses on just such a motivation. Its ideas are based on information from a unique source—the readings of Edgar Cayce. One of the foremost psychics of the twentieth century, Cayce gave the majority of his readings to individuals with health concerns who sought his advice. This source invites us to consider the whole person—spiritual, mental, and physical—as we work with our bodies. They take the perspective that our bodies are temples and should be cared for in that light: " . . . the love of and for a pure body is the most sacred experience in an entity's earthly sojourn . . . " (Edgar Cayce reading 436-2)[1] From this vantage point, working with weight control actually can represent a focused opportunity for growth.

To assist you with this goal, this booklet will help you address the patterns standing in your way—both

---

[1] The Edgar Cayce readings have each been assigned a two-part number for identification. The first digits indicate the specific number assigned to the topic or individual obtaining the reading. Since many received more than one reading, the second set of digits following the hyphen indicates the number in that particular series of readings.

behavioral and physiological. The Cayce readings indicate that excess weight results not only from an excess of starches in the diet, but also from an interplay of other factors. These include poor elimination patterns and an incoordination of the nervous system, which combined can produce a glandular imbalance, all leading to an altered metabolism of sugar. This booklet will provide you with suggestions in the areas of exercise, diet, and eliminations, and for coordinating the nervous and glandular systems to help you maintain physical balance. Additionally, our mental patterns of action and reaction will require special methods to reach and change them. Among other techniques, author Anne Hunt will guide you through the process of making your own pre-sleep suggestion tape.

Instead of calorie counting, this approach focuses on wellness and provides you with ideas and tools to help you on your journey to full health.

Eric A. Mein, M.D.
Meridian Institute

Dieting should not be so rigid as to appear that you can't do this or you can't do that, but rather let your attitude be that everything that is eaten, as well as every activity you undertake, be purposeful in conception, constructive in nature.

EDGAR CAYCE
PIONEER IN HOLISTIC HEALTH CARE

Chapter One

WHO NEEDS TO DIET?

DIETING IS SERIOUS BUSINESS

Weight loss is a serious and complex issue. It is not merely a question of excess pounds caused by excess calories. Diet and exercise are not simple solutions which can be applied universally for positive results. If you are overweight and have tried to trim both pounds and inches, you probably know firsthand the labyrinth which winds its way toward elusive success. You know all the false starts and dead ends. You've experienced them all before—maybe more than once.

Perhaps you've attacked your weight problem from so many angles for so many years that you're at the point of ultimate frustration. Even if your struggles have been short term, you probably have been wandering the labyrinth long enough to know that a clearer picture of where you're going and how to get there would be of immense help. That's what this book offers you.

WHAT MAKES THIS BOOK DIFFERENT

Weight No More is a complete program of weight loss based on an unusual source—the information given in the psychic readings of Edgar Cayce. This approach to weight loss embraces not only the physical, but the emotional and spiritual aspects as well. That's what makes it different from the hundreds of other weight-loss programs on the market. There's no calorie counting and no weighing in. Rather, you'll find a unique approach to examining what's behind your weight problem and learning to correct it using both mental and physical approaches and techniques. With persistency *and* consistency, this program can result in long-term success.

SETTING YOUR GOAL

Before embarking on any weight-loss program, it's important to take a good look in the mirror, literally and figuratively. To what image do you tend to compare yourself? Is the form of Bo Derek's perfect "10" body lurking somewhere in the back of your mind? Is Barbie so ingrained in your psyche that you've grown up to compare yourself to her dollish shape? Or perhaps it's Mel Gibson's physique that compels you to criticize your own?

These questions and concerns need to be dealt with in the early stages of your weight-loss plan. Do you need to lose ten pounds or thirty? What is *your* best weight? Try to get out of the habit of thinking that you need to fit into the "normal weight range" for people of your height, bone structure, and sex. If you have a chart that gives these weight ranges, throw it away. That will be your first positive step toward achieving a weight that is correct for you—not one that is right for someone *like you*.

The Cayce readings always stressed the uniqueness of the individual. This program of weight loss is geared toward helping you awaken to that uniqueness on all levels of your being. The result will be a happier, healthier, and fitter you.

ZEROING IN ON YOUR PROBLEM

If you have faced the problem of weight loss but have found only periodic success, then you know firsthand the complexity of the process. *You know that all weight problems are not the same.*

Below are four basic ways a weight problem can be experienced:

Fluctuating Weight Perhaps you've been up and down on the scales so often that you have motion sickness from the emotional highs and lows that accompany such a journey. And you'd give anything for a program that would even out this roller coaster ride once and for all. If this pattern describes you, then understanding the motives behind your ups and downs will be extremely important. It's highly likely that emotional issues also play a vital role in your struggles. Remember, your erratic diet and exercise levels can be extremely harmful and damaging to your body—not to mention your self-esteem.

Consistently Overweight On the other hand, you may be consistently overweight to the point that your excess pounds are a constant threat to your health and well-being. People who fall into this category truly need to find a program that will gradually bring their weight to within normal ranges. Though there are probably emotional factors which contribute to your problem, there may also be serious physiological imbalances which come into play. It's particularly important for people in this category to consult with their physician before they undertake any weight-loss program.

Cosmetically Overweight Some people have minor weight problems which potentially threaten only their opinion of themselves when they look in the mirror. People who fall into this category need to think first of increased activity as a way to trim down, complemented by a more healthful, lower-calorie diet.

Psychologically Overweight Some people merely "think" they are overweight, though to the outside world their shape is to be envied. If you fall into this category, you are suffering from the worst form of the Barbie-doll complex. Some image of perfection is so ingrained in your subconscious that your life may prove to be one needless diet after another. You need to find ways to lighten up on yourself, not on your diet!

DIET—TRULY A WAY OF LIFE

If you fall into any of the above categories, you'll find help in this book. What you will learn is a whole new way of looking at your life and shaping it for physical excellence. The result will be a more rewarding life style, a more positive self-image. In fact, the word "diet" actually comes from the Greek word *diaita*, which means "way of life." To the Greeks it was a creative thing, a way of creating beauty in body, mind, and spirit. It can and should be the same for you. That's what this book aims to help you accomplish.

Chapter Two

THE BODY, MIND, AND SPIRIT DIET

THE *WEIGHT NO MORE* APPROACH TO WEIGHT LOSS

The *Weight No More* program provides tools and guidelines to help you examine *your* unique struggles with excess weight. Understanding the origin of your weight problem is half the battle; the other half is taking that understanding and transforming it into a strategy for creating a new, healthful life style that fits your individual needs.

First, you'll learn how the Cayce readings viewed the harmony and interrelatedness of body, mind, and spirit. The interplay of these important aspects of ourselves is the cornerstone to understanding how we can become the best that we can be—spiritually, mentally, and physically.

Second, you'll look more closely at how mental patterns, attitudes, and emotions are affecting your success at weight control. You'll take a revealing quiz and begin to practice some mental exercises which can help you learn to flex your "mental muscle" to help trim those excess pounds.

Last, but not least, you'll look closely at how physical activities—ranging from diet and eliminations to exercise and special therapies—can be enlisted to help speed you on to success.

A CLOSER LOOK AT LIFE STYLE

All three of the above aspects in this weight-loss program deal ultimately with the way you live your life. Life style is a broad and all-encompassing concept and practice. In our society many have been taught to believe that life style is an outer thing, involving such items as the house we live in, the car we drive, where we vacation. The Cayce readings, however, paint a unique picture of how our lives are created, encompassing spiritual, mental, and physical energies. Time and again they state that we are composed of three distinct parts which combine to make a whole person—having a physical body, a mental body, and a spiritual body. In describing the relationship among these three bodies, the readings conveyed the following principle: "Spirit is the life, mind is the builder, and the physical is the result."

The bottom-line meaning of this statement is powerful. In many ways, it is the Cayce readings' formula for how the Life Force flows into the world and into our lives. Tapping into this Force in a positive way, allowing it to flow without hindrance through our bodies, is the key to success in correcting any physical problem. And excess weight is no exception.

As mentioned earlier, this program is designed to help you deal with your weight problem on all three of these levels—spirit, mind, and body. Here's a brief look at each one of these in turn.

SPIRIT IS THE LIFE

Within each of us is an innate wisdom that brings and renews life in our bodies. This reproductive energy is not relegated only to procreation but is involved daily on a cellular level, building and repairing our bodies. This energy or wisdom directs the complex operation of our bodies—in almost all cases without our conscious knowledge.

How is this wisdom transmitted to the physical body? There are specific points of contact between our spiritual and physical bodies. These conductors are our endocrine glands. The readings pay special attention to seven such glands in explaining the connection between the spiritual and the physical: the gonads, the cells of Leydig, the adrenals, the thymus, thyroid, pineal, and pituitary. These glands, along with the assistance of many other vital glands, secrete potent molecules which affect and regulate literally thousands of metabolic functions, including the regeneration of cells and tissues. They are all programmed, on a spiritual level, to function properly and to maintain health and balance within your body. You, after all, would be caught quite a bit short if you had to consciously direct your glands' activities.

Why, then, are our bodies not as perfect as the gods and goddesses of ancient Greece? Why are our bodies so individualized and of varying degrees of health and illness, if the Spirit which gives us life is of the same source and is perfect wisdom?

MIND IS THE BUILDER

Herein lies the rub. According to the Cayce readings, our mental bodies contain a collection of patterns which create our physical life. First, there are the genetic patterns and physiological tendencies which we chose on a mental level prior to birth. Tied in closely with these physiological tendencies is the "set point" theory which states that our bodies naturally gravitate to a particular weight. Throughout our lives we influence that "weight"—primarily by diet and exercise. Second, there are our conscious and subconscious mental patterns which are constantly shaping our lives and coming to bear on our inborn tendencies. These are most easily recognized as our attitudes and emotions.

If your attitudes and emotions result in a life of healthy, balanced meals and regular exercise, the physical result will be quite different than if you are inclined to the opposite. Likewise, if you live a life of great stress and negative thinking, without the tendency to employ constructive means to counteract the effects of this pressure, there will be unpleasant effects on your body and your health.

It is very important to understand that our attitudes and emotions and the mental patterns which create them are deeply ingrained in our being. We all know from our past experiences that we cannot simply say to ourselves "No more ice cream for me" or "I'm going to take a one-mile walk every day" and consider our life style changed. A conscious decision often has little effect on our patterns of behavior. Life would be much simpler if it did.

What, then, are mental patterns? Where do they originate? How can they be changed?

The subconscious mind houses much of our awareness. It is here that mental patterns play out their agendas, most often completely hidden from us. They come from many complex sources. One catalyst can be how we were treated as children, perhaps by a parent, a sibling, a friend, a teacher. Another is the kind of media we were exposed to while growing up. From Barbie dolls to Twiggy we were taught that slim and trim is desirable, anything less (or should we say more?) is unattractive. The list of subconscious motivators and de-motivators could go on and on.

Changing these patterns is an important element in healing the body in general; specifically, it is the key to weight loss. If you've struggled with weight control for any period of time, you know by now that it is a complex issue. You know that it's not simply *what* you eat, for if it was you could easily change that and all would be well. It's also *why* you eat, *why* you snack, *why* you can't stay on an exercise routine that is important. What you need are tools to change the subconscious mind. Beyond even that you need to know what patterns have to be changed and into what you need to change them. This book will help you in all these areas.

PHYSICAL IS THE RESULT

The body you see in your mirror is a result of your mental patterns and how they have affected your body's physiology.

But where exactly are these patterns stored? In the approximately 70 trillion cells that make up your body! How these cells are nurtured and allowed to function is the key to health and fitness. They need to receive the right signals from your mind or mental body, they need to exist in an environment free of toxins, and they need to receive the proper nutrition. If they are given these three elements, they can slowly but surely begin to realize the perfection that gives them life. According to Cayce, careful, healthful work on both a mental and physical level can help influence these patterns and their physiological results in the direction you want them to go—which is toward greater health and wholeness.

HONOR YOUR BODY

You will be most successful if your ultimate goal in this diet is to honor your body and seek for it the ultimate in balance and health. Marvel at its ability to regulate its every activity. Set as your highest purpose a desire to create an ideal environment in which the Life Force can flow and heal. Include in your goal an intent to use your body to do good service in the world. And success will be virtually yours.

Chapter Three

HOW TO GET STARTED

LAUNCHING FOR SUCCESS

Most weight-loss books begin with a discussion of your body's physiology, from the role of metabolism to the pros and cons of the ketonic state (depending upon what diet you're reading about!). If you've read these books and tried these diets, you know that they are often the first leg of a journey to nowhere. In fact, recent statistics indicate that 85% of the people who diet and lose weight, gain it back. So, if you've been there before, you're in a multitude of company.

One of the reasons people gain this weight back is that they haven't been able to understand and deal with completely all the factors that come into play in their unique problem. Dieters know that there is something missing in almost every diet, though the identity of that something is a vague mystery. Some feel that it is a physiological imbalance. Others feel that there are complex emotional issues involved. The list goes on and on.

The truth is that there are truly dozens of possible causes behind any and all weight problems. You are about to begin an exploration of what those real, bottom-line causes might be.

SAMPLE SYNDROMES

Let's examine for a moment some typical scenarios that revolve around weight-loss issues. You'll be able to see at once that more factors are at play than a simple decision to lose weight for personal well-being. Feelings are involved. Motives. And desires.

The "Get-in-Shape-for-the-Beach" Syndrome

In February Mary promised herself that by June 1 she'd be slim and in shape for the beach. But work was hectic during the intervening months and interfered with her diet and exercise program. When May 15 rolled around, Mary had put on even more weight. Now, she's in the market for any book that promises a 14-day weight-loss program. And she'll do just about anything to succeed.

The "He-Wants-Me-Thin-but-They-Want Me-Fat" Syndrome

A month ago Nancy's husband made a casual comment about her weight that hurt her feelings. She decided to go on a diet immediately. Then, her family began to complain about the low-calorie evening fare. They liked meals the way they used to be. Nancy became discouraged and quit. "They can't have their cake and eat it, too" became her self-defeating motto.

The "Impossible-Comparison" Syndrome

January 5 is Rose and Bill's 30th wedding anniversary. Bill has just announced a surprise Christmas trip to Hawaii to celebrate. Rose already begins to feel self-conscious about her weight next to those shapely native girls doing the hula. It's November 15 now and a maze of holiday dinner events, parties, and "too cold to exercise" weather stand between her and dieting success. Bill can't understand Rose's glum mood after the initial delight at his thoughtfulness.

These scenarios are merely a sampling of the kinds of challenges a dieter meets. Events such as these are very discouraging. On some level, they make you feel that weight control is useless. How can you even begin the battle of the bulge—much less win it—with odds such as these?

What exactly are the odds? Not enough time. Temptation. Predetermined defeat. Family intervention. Comparison with others. These and many other similar odds are common and very real in the weight-loss battle. But there is something very interesting about these scenarios that can help you understand your struggles more fully and begin to position yourself to succeed.

In each of the cases above, the stimulus to lose weight *appears* to be from an outer source and the roadblock to success *seems* to come from external pressures or circumstances as well. The "dieter" appears to be trying to make other people happy—whether they're strangers on the beach who see you walk by or your adoring husband who you suddenly feel may prefer a native dancing girl to his wife of 30 years.

Paint a picture in your head of a scenario in your life in which weight loss became a looming issue. Examine it closely. Had you, like the three women above, unconsciously set yourself up for defeat? Has your dieting life been full of other similar "Waterloos"?

PURPOSES AND REASONS

On the surface, our purposes for desiring to lose weight would probably sound very similar to the scenarios above. There would be different circumstances and different players, but the stories would sound quite similar. We would feel some purpose for needing to lose weight, perhaps for an upcoming special event or in response to a doctor's direct orders.

Our reasons for failure also appear similar. Dieting is inconvenient. We aren't getting the results we want fast enough. We're afraid we'll die of malnourishment long before we reach our dieting goals!

MOTIVES AND PATTERNS

Beneath these purposes and reasons lurk the true challenges in our ongoing struggles: motivations and patterns. Motivations are often seeded in the subconscious mind and are powerful forces in our lives. They are the impulse that sets us on a particular course. As we travel along that course, we fall into patterns—sometimes of success, other times of failure.

Whenever we undertake a weight-loss program, it is likely that there are several motives coming into play. *Motives compel you to begin a diet; patterns determine your level of success.*

Is there a way to determine motives? Can patterns be identified? The following quiz may shed some light on these questions:

MOTIVES AND PATTERNS QUIZ

For each of the items on the questionnaire below, select the answer that best describes you. If you find that more than one answer is equally true of you in any given question, circle both. If none of the answers in a given question is at all descriptive of you, simply leave that item unanswered.

1. I'm most likely to start a weight-loss program when:
a. I want to look better for some special occasion that's just around the corner.
b. I'm feeling confident and in control of my life.
c. I catch an unguarded glimpse of myself in a mirror and hate what I see.
d. My regular home and work responsibilities are lightened or suspended in some way.
e. There are the fewest food-oriented occasions on my upcoming calendar.

2. I am most comfortable (or least uncomfortable) with my body when:
a. The cooler seasons allow me to hide it in bulky clothes.

b. I can find slenderizing clothing styles to wear.
c. I am with other people who like to eat a lot and make no apologies about it.
d. The scale, clothing sizes, tape measurements, etc., are at the very lowest or smallest that have ever been in my adult life.
e. I am with people who are at least as overweight as I am.

3. When I abandon a weight-loss program, it's usually because:
a. I don't get the results I want as quickly as I expect them.
b. The results I get don't seem to improve my appearance very much.
c. I'm disappointed to find that whenever I'm thinner I'm less happy in some ways than I was with my old life style.
d. It's just too difficult to fit diet and/or exercise programs around my family and job responsibilities.
e. I feel I'm missing too many food-centered good times.

4. When I have been doing fairly well on a weight-loss program and then enter a stressful period in my life, I'm most likely to:
a. Feel guilty over the negative impact my diet and/or exercise efforts have been making on others (i.e., time away from family, lack of "lovin' from the oven," etc.).
b. Decide that I am coping poorly because I am not getting enough to eat and/or enough physical relaxation time.
c. Blame myself for the troubles in my life and eat in a self-destructive frame of mind.
d. Work so hard at alleviating the stressful conditions that there really isn't enough time left for weight-loss efforts.
e. Feel discouraged about everything and think "what's the use?" and give up on my weight-loss program.

5. I feel that I am/would be most attractive physically when:
a. One or more aspects of my basic body structure or facial features are dramatically altered (beyond what weight loss would accomplish).
b. My weight is at or below the lowest point in the normal range for my height.

c. I am wearing an expensive new outfit.

d. I receive embarrassing but flattering attentions from the opposite sex.

e. I am around people who are significantly more overweight than I am and don't seem to be worried about it.

6. When I'm feeling especially unattractive, my tendency is to:
a. Devote more energy to pleasing my family and/or colleagues.
b. Compare myself unfavorably with slim and attractive public personalities.
c. Feel insignificant and invisible.
d. Think that everyone is noticing how unattractive I look.
e. Blame it on being too busy to take proper care of myself.

7. During the first week of dieting, my feelings about my weight-loss attempts are best described as:
a. A sense of self-consciousness about what others may be thinking about my progress.
b. A feeling that my efforts are probably being wasted because they have always failed in the past.
c. Impatience about how slow my progress seems to be.
d. Fear that I'll go off my diet during the upcoming weekend.
e. Concern that my limited food intake may make me more susceptible to becoming ill.

8. If I dramatically depart from my diet routine one day, my reaction is most likely to be:
a. A crash diet for the next day or two.
b. A feeling that I deserved a good meal because of the hard work I put in that week.
c. Reconsideration of whether I really needed to be dieting at all.
d. A feeling that I did the right thing by eating what was put in front of me rather than make a fuss and ask for something special.
e. A feeling that people are talking about my lack of willpower behind my back.

9. When I include an exercise routine as a part of my weight-loss program, it usually ends up this way:

a. I stick with it for several days until I feel that work or other special projects are falling behind.

b. I compare myself unfavorably to others who are exercising, then I become discouraged and quit.

c. I feel as though I'm not spending enough time with my loved ones and/or friends, so I gradually get out of my routine in favor of more time with them.

d. I pull a muscle or strain my back and need to quit.

e. I work out hard for two or three weeks and then become discouraged that my efforts don't have the dramatic results for which I had hoped.

10. Overall, my struggle with weight has caused me the *most* unhappiness because:

a. Eating is one of the things I enjoy most in life.

b. My efforts to control my weight lead to conflicts with family members and friends who are unconvinced or feel left behind when I try to change my life style.

c. I've been disappointed to find that each time I've lost weight my problems seem as bad as or even worse than ever.

d. I have never felt "normal" or as good as other people.

e. My attempts to control my weight have been repeated experiences of failure to attain or maintain my goals.

SCORING

STEP ONE: Circle the letter-number pairs for each of the answers below that corresponds to the *letters* of the answers you chose in questions 1-10 above. For example, if your response to question #1 was "c," then you'll circle "c" and "4":

C
4

3. a b c d e   4. a b c d e
    5 4 3 2 1   2 3 4 1 5

5. a b c d e   6. a b c d e
    4 5 1 3 2   2 5 3 4 1

7. a b c d e   8. a b c d e
    2 4 5 1 3   5 1 3 2 4

9. a b c d e   10. a b c d e
    1 4 2 3 5   1 2 3 4 5

STEP TWO: Count up the number of times your circled letter-number pairs included each of the following numbers:

1's   7
2's   4
3's   7
4's   6
5's   8

WHAT YOUR ANSWERS MEAN

It is significant if your answers tended to cluster around one or two of the above numbers. Any number that popped up three or more times is particularly significant and revealing. The possible answers to all of the questions above are designed to tie into particular archetypes of motivation which may be coming into play in your struggles with weight control. You may find that you have a tendency toward several different types. If you do, you're not alone. Remember, weight control is a complex issue and you are a complex being.

Type 1. The Gourmet If you had a surplus of 1's in your answers, it probably means that weight control is really not your number one priority. There are things in life which you enjoy and feel responsibility toward which come before your desires to trim down. A nice evening out at a gourmet restaurant may be one. You may need to modify your diet and behavior between social events so that you can consume those extra calories (guilt-free!) when they are placed ceremoniously before you. If you aren't obese and your health is good, your best strategy may be to stay just the way you are.

Type 2. The Pleaser If you tended toward 2's, it's likely that the priorities and demands of others shape your outlook and actions regarding weight loss. Family pressures and responsibilities or long hours at work cut into your routine and make it difficult for you to stay on any program. You need to examine ways to reconcile your needs with the needs of others. Compromise may be in order, but the days of complete surrender need to be put behind you.

Type 3. The Protector If 3's are prominent in your answers, it's likely that you feel you need weight to buffer you from the outside world. Though you think you want to lose weight, you may actually feel more comfortable and secure with excess pounds. Insecurity and lack of self-confidence may be at the root of your problem. You need to look for ways to bolster your security and confidence.

Type 4. The Critic If 4's pop up frequently in your responses, poor self-image may be at the root of your problem. Unlike the 3's, you are not putting on extra pounds to protect yourself but rather to sabotage yourself. Deep down inside, you are your own greatest critic. You probably don't feel worthy of looking and feeling good. You need to look for ways to build self-esteem.

Type 5. The Perfectionist If 5's are plentiful in your answers, unrealistic goals may be your greatest enemy. Just as the perfectionist requires that every little detail be in order, you zero in on any sign of a single excess pound. Are you really cut out to be a swimsuit model? Are you demanding too much of yourself? It may be time to re-examine your desire to lose weight. At the very least, you need to re-examine the goals you set, both in terms of pounds and of days. Relax.

WRAPPING UP

Look back at the scenarios described at the beginning of this chapter. Though we can't take the "Motives and Patterns Quiz" for these three women, we can make certain observations about each of them. In short, it's obvious that Mary wants to be "perfect" for the beach at all costs. Nancy wants to "please" her family regardless of her personal needs. And Rose's major concern is the thought of having to abstain from "gourmet" holiday meals in preparation for her anniversary trip.

WHAT DOES ALL THIS MEAN?

Getting a handle on your motives for embarking upon a weight-loss program is vital for ultimate success. Inherent in motives are all the stumbling blocks for defeat. Motives are inner drives—what we can't necessarily see or recognize readily on a conscious level. They are often embedded in our subconscious. Thus they create results; often not what we had in mind. Yet they have a tremendous effect on the results of our activities.

If you discovered that you are a "Critic," you may be wondering where you go for self-esteem? If you are a "Pleaser," how can you put other people's needs and expectations aside?

Start by continuing with this book. You'll find suggestions for beginning where you are to reprogram some of the motivational patterns which stand between you and success.

ATTITUDES ABOUT YOURSELF CREATE WHO YOU ARE

Reflect for a moment on the Cayce readings' concept of "mind is the builder." In simple terms, it means that your mind has created not only your body but also the circumstances in which you find yourself. For the most part, this "creating" has happened on a subconscious level. Your subconscious mind is a powerful reserve which should be programmed for happiness and success.

Chapter Four

MENTAL MUSCLE

BEGIN WITH THE END

It's time to begin enlisting the power of your mind to start you on the road to weight-loss success. The following exercise is a first step in planting a positive image of yourself in your subconscious. It involves imaging what you wish to be the lasting result of your weight-loss efforts.

Exercise One
THE IDEAL YOU

Take out a sheet of paper and pen or pencil. Retreat to a quiet place where there will be no interruptions. Now, take a few minutes to imagine what your goals are for weight loss and physical improvement. Paint a picture of yourself in your mind, one that is optimum *and* realistic for your body structure and appearance. Be thankful for the image that you see and how it expresses your uniqueness.

Think also about your inner spiritual and emotional being. How will you feel about yourself and about others? Here is a good place to create positive thoughts to replace the possible feelings of low self-esteem or overly zealous perfectionism you may have discovered in your motivational quiz. Paint a picture of the best you, who is full of love for all creation.

Now, imagine what your activities will be like when you have reached your goal. Choose an average day, during which you will go about your daily routine, one which includes a healthful diet and healthful activities. Don't feel constrained by your current habits and patterns. Those are what you want to change. Make this day an ideal day in your ideal body.

Now, write down your thoughts. Start with a detailed description of how you look and how you feel. Then, begin in the morning and describe the day as it unfolds. Include in your day some of what you will do with your renewed, healthful body.

After you've finished writing, put this paper aside for a few days. Later, pull it out again and redo it, repeating the process—perhaps refining some points, perhaps leaving others as you first imagined them. Go over what you've written several times over a period of a month or two, as you begin to shape your new healthful life style. Create this paper so that it reflects what you are working for and how you will use your body for your own good and the good of others.

Once you feel that your ideal you and ideal day are exactly as you want them, put the paper away somewhere out of sight, perhaps in a desk drawer. What you have done is use your imagination and concentration to set positive, constructive thoughts in motion. Those thoughts are now planted in your subconscious and will work to assist you in your new life-style plan.

Many people who have done an exercise such as this have found that this piece of paper often pops up a year or more later. Remarkably, many report that the day which they had earlier described has come to fruition.

Exercise Two
PRE-SLEEP SUGGESTION

The Cayce readings suggested another powerful, useful, and effective method for implanting positive, constructive thoughts in the subconscious to help bring about positive change. Just prior to your going to sleep, the readings indicated that the subconscious mind is most accessible. Using "pre-sleep" suggestions can gently persuade your mind to build a foundation of positive thoughts upon which to build your new life style.

How can you make use of pre-sleep suggestion to lose weight? One easy way is to turn to Appendix C and learn how to obtain a prerecorded pre-sleep tape geared toward weight loss.

Another way is to record your own tape—a task which is much easier than it may sound. Begin by reading through the following script to become familiar with it. Feel free to modify it to make it more personalized for you. Follow only one rule in making these minor changes—make sure that any words or phrases you substitute are positive and uplifting. Once you are comfortable with your script, sit down with a tape recorder and record, using a soothing, slowly paced voice, and pausing approximately 10 seconds between phrases (indicated by " . . . ") and sentences. You might wish to have soothing music playing in the background to provide a backdrop to your voice. This tape with its affirmations will be food for your subconscious mind. Positive thoughts are one form of nourishment that is never restricted.

As you practice the script, notice that the positive thoughts are oriented to address the archetypal patterns discussed earlier. This script will help repattern you for more positive motivational responses.

You will gain the optimum benefit from this tape by listening to it on a nightly basis just while you are going to sleep. For best results play the tape at a soothing and comfortable volume near your bedside. If you have a cassette player that will play both sides of a tape consecutively, you may want to record the script on each side so that it can play twice as long without interruption. Most important, make sure the tape is set up so that it will turn off automatically.

PRE-SLEEP TAPE SCRIPT
(to be read aloud onto cassette tape)

It's time to close your eyes now ... to rest and relax and enjoy the peacefulness of sleeping. Focus on your breathing, allowing yourself to breathe in deeply and exhale completely. Feel the relaxation your rhythmic breathing brings to your body. With each breath in, you are supplying your body with a bounty of fresh, life-giving air ... with each breath out, you are helping your body release stale air and the worries of the day. You are becoming

more and more relaxed with each progressive breath. Breathe in
... breathe out ... breathe in ... breathe out ... breathe in ...
breathe out. You are becoming more and more relaxed with
each passing moment ... more and more a part of your body. You
are at one with your body ... and aware of how good and peaceful it feels. You are opening to new ways of seeing your life ...
your mind is opening to positive suggestion. You feel good about
your life and the way it is transforming each day ... toward a better you ... a healthier and more fulfilled you. You are unique. You
are loved. You are a special part of God's creation ... God loves
you and is with you in your life. God supports you as you grow
more and more in God's love. You are a part of humanity. Others
love you for who you are and who you are becoming. Feel this
love. Feel the love you have for yourself ... the true love that is a
part of your being ... the love that understands you and embraces you ... and accepts you for who you are. Let this love
grow and multiply ... you are like a seed planted in spring that
grows and reaches to the sun, becoming stronger and more
beautiful with time ... you are loved by all of creation ... you are a
part of all creation. You want to be the best that you can be ... to
reach and stretch toward your highest purpose. You are gentle
with yourself and respect and love your uniqueness. God and
others love your uniqueness. With each day it becomes easier
and easier to eat a balanced diet ... you are eating the foods that
your body needs. It is easier to drink the water your body needs
... you feel it cleansing and washing every cell of your body. With
each day you have more energy ... you feel a little bit lighter ...
you are coming closer and closer to your ideal body. You are
using this body to help others. Your lighter, healthier body is of
more and more service ... there are many people you have much
to give to. You have balanced, loving relationships ... you are in
touch with your feelings ... you know your needs ... and you trust
that they will be satisfied. There is a bounty of all that you need
available to you. Your body is your friend and your home ... it

brings you joy. Floating into your mind is a positive memory of how your body let you do something wonderful... some beautiful feeling or event that your body let you experience. The memory is gradually taking shape. You know that your body is your best friend... this memory reminds you of the many gifts your body has given you... it brings you joy and pleasure. Your body wants to be healthy and happy... it wants and desires healthful foods. You treat it as you would any good friend... you give it nourishment and love. It is easier to exercise... with each day you love the feeling of exercise more and more. You treat your body well... your body feels vital and alive... you have renewed energy. You feel lighter and lighter. Your life is full of purpose. As you grow lighter, something good is happening... you are being healed. You are thankful for the chance to feel this new lightness... you are learning new things about your body... it is your friend. You are becoming a better and better person as you become lighter... you feel better... your mind is more at ease... you are more sensitive and understanding. You have a new life style... if you feel empty... you drink water... or eat a healthful meal that is just what your body needs. Every cell in your body is thanking you... every day is a wonderful new experience. All the cells in your body are new friends... they contribute to your success... they support you. You desire what your body needs... you are aware of your true needs... you meet your needs in healthy ways. You have a new freedom... you enjoy what you eat and it is good for you. You feel good about your meals... each day it is easier and easier to eat what you really need. You are closer and closer to your ideal weight... you are freer... you are lighter. You are patient with your progress... you enjoy the gradual growing... you enjoy every step along the way. You are aware of the beauty of each day... of the marvelous world you live in... you know lasting results are happening... Your mind is drifting gently into a natural, comfortable sleep... a place where you are safe and at peace. You are being carried into sleep as if on gentle, rolling waves ... waves that caress your body ... your feelings ... and your soul ... You may hear your inner voice whispering all the positive feelings you have about your body ... they sound good to you ... your body feels good to you ... it is a pleasant home for your soul ... it is your friend. [End of script]

Exercise Three
DAILY JOURNAL

A daily journal is a way of tracking your progress and making sure that you consciously evaluate, without being overly critical, your activities in terms of the program you have set for yourself. It is important that this journal be an exercise in introspection, not self-criticism. Your feeling upon completing each entry should be the satisfaction of having taken one more step toward success—even if the "step" was evaluating some of the reasons why you may have temporarily gotten away from your plan.

When you sit down to make your daily entries, ask yourself the following questions:

> How did I do on my new life-style plan today?
> If I did well, what circumstances surrounded my success?
> If I departed a bit from my plan, what factors or influences may have come into play?
> How do I feel about my overall progress (ask this question weekly, rather than daily)?

Be sure to include any other feelings and insights that you think are relevant. Then, review your journal every two or three weeks. What you want to look for are patterns which seem to result in success and patterns which seem to slow your progress. Evaluate both types of patterns and do three things.

First, repeat the things you did which resulted in a deeper feeling of self-esteem. Perhaps taking the time in the morning to read the newspaper gave you a feeling of being in touch with current events. When you were able to join in a conversation about the economy with knowledge and understanding, you felt confident and insightful. Your self-esteem and self-image were given a nudge in a positive direction. Look for the possibility that you stuck to your diet plan more closely when you were also doing things which improved your thoughts and feelings about yourself.

Second, create more positive circumstances which seem to herald success. For instance, if a trip to a farmer's market on Saturday seems to have resulted in healthier meals all week long, then make the trip to the farmer's market a Saturday ritual. Or, if finding a friend to join you on an evening walk gave you the added push to get out the door, see if you can find a walking buddy who's as serious about his or her program as you are.

Third, try to plan around the kinds of events which seem to tempt you adversely. If rushing off to work without packing a lunch results in a mad dash through a fast-food place, begin to pack your lunch the night before. Or, if you find that your urges for a sweet treat drive you to a package of cookies that you munch on for days, consider going out for an ice cream cone instead. The cone will satisfy your taste buds without lingering as a temptation in the cupboard.

WILLPOWER

The word *willpower* was bound to come up eventually. What respectable diet book would fail to introduce this elusive character at least in passing? But there's good news. The Cayce perspective on the will is so unique that you will probably learn something new—and useful—in your weight-loss strategy.

Ultimate success with any diet requires the cooperation of the will. All individuals have wills of their own. There is no such thing as someone who lacks this personal power. In fact, it is the same will that leads you down the path to overeating that can turn you on to the path of dietary self-control. Hard to believe? Look at it this way. According to Cayce, the soul has three attributes: pure energy, the mind which creates patterns to shape the energy, and the will which directs how the creative mind works. You can use your will to realize your spiritual nature by seeking to align it with your highest ideals, or you can use it for more destructive purposes. It is the great individualizer. The freedom of your will makes you unique. The will is the factor behind your choices, the architect of your patterns. It can be brought under your control and used to bring your body and spirit into alignment and health.

Exericse Four
WILLPOWER MUSCLE BUILDERS

Believe it or not, aligning your will with a more constructive life style is possible. Refreshingly, the following exercise in directing your will has nothing to do with dieting.

Many diets will simply say "Use your willpower" to drink this diet shake while everyone else at the office goes out for a pizza. "Summon it up and put it to work," the diet plan will admonish. But this approach can often lead to frustration. Since most of us on a conscious level are relatively strangers to our will, it can be quite difficult to enter into a partnership with it. To begin to understand your will, play with the following exercise for a week or two:

In the course of your daily routine begin to recognize opportunities to summon up your willpower to make what you *know to be* the right decision.

For instance, as you're driving home from the office and you notice that your gas tank is on empty, observe your inner dialogue. "I know I ought to get gas now, but I'm exhausted. I just want to get home. I can stop in the morning or tomorrow at lunch." What this decision often leads to is frustration. You get a late start for the office the next day, so you have to bypass the station. Then, everyone goes out for lunch so you catch a ride with an office mate, leaving your "on empty" car behind. That night, on your way home, you're right back where you were the night before.

This scenario unfolds, albeit wearing different disguises, thousands of times in the course of our lives.

To break this pattern, begin to see these as opportunities to exercise your will. First, promise yourself that you'll choose what you feel to be the right action approximately one out of two or three times. With time, try to make more and more correct choices. But don't, under any circumstances, engage in self-criticism when you make a mistake. This may take willpower in itself! Simply pick yourself up, and begin anew with the next challenge.

Kinds of opportunities that might arise:
>   Take the trash out tonight, not tomorrow
>   Choose fresh vegetables, rather than canned
>   Take a morning walk, instead of a second cup of coffee

When you are in the process of making a decision, observe how you feel during the process. If it is a "painful" decision, something you really don't want to know or to do, you might feel as though the mental process involved almost gives you a headache. But when you make the right decision and motivate yourself to move in the right direction, you might notice a subtle or even more pronounced feeling at the base of your throat. According to Cayce, the thyroid gland is how the spiritual aspect of the will is channeled into the physical plane.

Try to become familiar with the feeling that success gives you. With time, it becomes easier to make the right choices because you come to desire this positive, uplifting feeling. The next step will be to apply this exercise to your diet and body therapy program.

Chapter Five

BUILDING A HEALTHIER BODY

The inner exploration you have engaged in up to this point has prepared you to begin a diet and therapy program that will provide your body with the life-giving energies it needs to reach its full potential.

FACTORS THAT CONTRIBUTE TO EXCESS WEIGHT

The Cayce readings indicated four primary physiological factors which contribute to a tendency toward excess weight:

Incorrect diet

Poor eliminations and assimilation

Incoordination of the nervous systems

Glandular imbalance

GETTING THE MOST OUT OF WHAT YOU EAT

It's important to get the most out of what you eat. In fact, many dietitians believe that your body's nutritional needs come into play in creating your appetites. You will have an appetite until your body's nutritional needs are met. This makes sense. We know that the body is innately wise. All cells know their nutritional needs. They will call for their needs in the form of appetite until their hunger is satisfied. If you are eating empty calories, your body will still call for more food, until it gets what it needs. Hand in hand with the importance of what you put in your mouth is your body's ability to assimilate or process that food.

You see, diet is simply what you eat. Nutrition is what happens to the food after you eat it. Assimilation is how your body through its complex metabolic processes is able to use the food. If any of these processes are out of whack, your body is likely to call for more food. Then the real problems begin.

ELIMINATIONS

To prepare the physical body for dieting success, it is wise to get the body ready to assimilate food properly. The five major elimination organs are the kidneys, colon, liver, skin, and lungs. These are the key players in this strategy. If they are not properly functioning, a toxic buildup in the system results.

Your body is called upon to dispose of many different

kinds of waste on a daily basis. They are, of course, the byproducts of the foods you eat—including the additives and preservatives which are plentiful in much of what you consume. Also, there are the pollutants that are taken into your system through your lungs, not to mention chemicals that come in through the skin. These additions are compounded then with internally generated wastes. Energy is burned and creates waste byproducts. Believe it or not, billions of cells die each day, and all of this material must be removed from your body to allow for an optimum level of assimilation.

Here's an outline of your body's elimination systems plus therapeutic suggestions for keeping them in order.

KIDNEYS AND LIVER

According to the Cayce readings, the kidneys actually function in an equal partnership with the liver. Both organs process the blood, filtering it for wastes and preparing the wastes for disposal. Any imbalance between these two organs can overwork one of the two and risk the possibility of toxins being thrown back into the system. The best routine to follow to keep the kidneys and liver healthy and effective is to drink six to eight glasses of pure (preferably spring) water a day. This practice will also benefit the colon and the skin.

Here's a suggested routine which will help you to pace yourself to drink this amount of water daily. Note that Cayce recommended that your first half glass of water in the morning be warm because it will help cleanse a relatively empty colon after the nighttime fast.

When	Glasses
Upon arising (warm)	½
Mid-morning and afternoon	2
Before breakfast, lunch, and dinner	3
After breakfast, lunch, and dinner	3
Total	8½

Are you concerned that this excess water will result in water retention and thus add more pounds? Put this thought aside, now and forever. Water is vital to life and is vital in the proper functioning of your entire body. Water is the primary conductor of removal of wastes from your body. Without enough water, wastes build up. A buildup of wastes can actually result in retention of the water that is in your system.

COLON

Besides consuming an ample supply of water each and every day, be sure to include a substantial amount of fiber in your diet. When you read about the "Weight No More Diet" in the next chapter, you'll see that it is a high-fiber approach to sound nutrition. Supplement this diet with natural laxatives, such as figs and raisins, and your colon will benefit.

An occasional colonic by a professional therapist or a self-administered enema will also be of benefit. A periodic internal cleansing of the colon makes sense. No matter how fibrous your diet or how consistent you are in your intake of water, there will be a buildup of wastes clinging to the walls and hiding in the folds of the colon.

What if you can't find someone from whom you can

receive a colonic? Then administer an enema to yourself at home. Though a colonic is as effective as receiving four to six enemas, an internal cleansing of either kind, carefully administered, will have tremendous effects on your health.

See Appendix D for directions on administering an enema.

There's also a special Cayce readings' therapy which is recommended to stimulate the liver, gall bladder, and colon. It is one of the most unique therapies suggested in the readings: the castor oil pack. The use of this pack, applied externally, was recommended in literally hundreds of Cayce readings. The specific benefit this therapy can have on the individual wishing to lose weight is that it can help improve assimilation through improved eliminations.

Refer to Appendix D for instructions on how to prepare and apply a castor oil pack.

LUNGS

Fresh air and deep breathing are the cornerstones of healthy eliminations through the lungs. Here's an exercise to wake up your lungs in the morning.

Upon arising, stand in front of an open window (the air outside, we hope, would be fresh!) and breathe deeply. Gradually raise your hands and arms above your head; at the same time rise up on your toes and stretch your leg muscles. Then, with a flowing motion, bend forward from the hips (this takes balance and practice!), exhaling through the nose. After your lungs are empty, inhale through the mouth and straighten up. Repeat for five to six minutes. Continue with your breathing exercise by closing first your right nostril with your right forefinger, then raise your left arm above your head and breathe in deeply through the left nostril. Exhale through the mouth and lower your arm. Repeat in the same way, this time closing your left nostril and breathing in deeply through your right, raising your right arm. Exhale through your mouth and lower your arm.

SKIN

Perspiration is an important elimination process in general and has particular benefit to the skin. Any exercise you engage in that produces perspiration is doing your elimination systems a world of good.

Another way of increasing perspiration is to take a steam bath. The best place for obtaining a steam bath to promote a thorough cleansing through perspiration is in a health facility that provides this service. Many massage therapists, for instance, will have a steam cabinet available so that you could take a steam before your massage. Also, you may belong to a health club that provides a steam room. If you do, don't overlook the benefit of a good steam, for five to ten minutes, after your workout.

But steams aren't relegated to only the fortunate few who have access to such facilities. Hydrotherapy can also be administered at home. See Appendix D for directions on how to take a home steam bath.

Another excellent stimulant for the skin and the eliminations in general is massage. This form of therapy builds superficial circulation in the skin and muscles which facilitates loosening toxic buildup so that it can be eliminated. Seek out a local massage therapist who can provide you with a steam and massage to give you the optimum benefits.

INCOORDINATION OF THE NERVOUS SYSTEM

Incoordination of the nervous system was also flagged as a possible factor in weight problems. The readings identified three major components of the nervous system: the cerebrospinal, the autonomic, and the sensory systems. Incoordination of the cerebrospinal and autonomic systems was pinpointed several times in the readings as an element which contributed to a tendency toward obesity. Combined with poor eliminations, any disparity among these systems can result in a glandular imbalance which adversely disturbs the metabolism.

The cerebrospinal nervous system consists of the brain and spinal cord, which operate under voluntary control. If you choose to go for a walk, lift a box, or write a letter to a friend, you enlist the support of your cerebrospinal system. The autonomic nervous system, of which the sympathetic and parasympathetic systems are a part, operates largely involuntarily.

Let's look at just one aspect of the autonomic system: the sympathetic system whose importance is often underestimated. It consists of two chains of nerves that run along each side of the spine. This system directs the activities of the organs and glands, stimulates and controls blood vessels, and helps coordinate the immune system. The Cayce readings indicate that through this system the mind, carrying subconscious and soul forces, communicates with the body. Thus, this system relays our mental patterns to the cells of the physical body.

What are the possible results of an imbalance of these systems? Mixed messages and poor communication. What happens is that our bodily functions can go haywire. Eliminations are affected. Organ functions become less than optimal. And our metabolic processes, so central to weight control, become imbalanced.

How can you coordinate your nervous systems? The best route is to find an osteopath or chiropractor with whom you feel comfortable discussing your weight problem. Let him or her know your goals and enlist this professional assistance to help you reach them.

The spinal adjustments your doctor administers will be aimed toward correcting any spinal misalignments. These misalignments can cause a disruption of the nerve impulses in both the cerebrospinal and the sympathetic nervous system. A correctly aligned spine will definitely help to straighten your road to success.

GLANDULAR IMBALANCE

The Cayce readings zeroed in on glandular imbalance as a possible factor contributing to excess weight. Although most diet programs target the thyroid gland as a major player in the regulation of metabolism, Cayce also included other glands and glandular tissues as being involved in proper weight control. As discussed in Chapter Two, the glands release potent molecules or hormones which regulate the body's vast and complex metabolic functions. Thus, an imbalance in this area can have an incredible impact on your body's ability to regulate its weight.

ROLE OF METABOLISM

What exactly is metabolism? In simple terms, it is the process by which your body assimilates food and builds up energy (anabolism), and then expends and breaks down that energy (catabolism). When anabolism exceeds catabolism, your body gains. When the opposite is true, your body loses.

Your metabolic rate is the rate at which your body burns fuel when resting. It is different for each of us and can vary throughout our lifetime. A slow metabolic rate requires less fuel, a fast metabolic rate requires more.

RESTORING GLANDULAR BALANCE

The Cayce readings often recommended the use of Atomidine (iodine trichloride) to help restore glandular balance. A standard routine is a five-day series. On the first day, take one drop in half a glass of water. On the second day, two drops. On the third, three drops. The fourth day go back down to two drops and on the fifth day only one drop. Repeat this five-day cycle every 28 days.

Chapter Six

CAN-DO DIET AND EXERCISE TIPS

BUT WHAT CAN I EAT?

Any dieter, seasoned or not, is wondering by now what foods are included on this diet. The answer is "Almost all." Now we're ready for the second question: How much can I eat? "All that you need."

You'll be glad to know that the Cayce readings encouraged the enjoyment of nutritious, balanced meals. "Take *time* to eat and to eat the right thing . . . " (Edgar Cayce reading 243-23) was one way the readings put it. Your diet should be well balanced among all of nature's bountiful and healthful foods.

Many of the diets popular today are as far from this kind of common-sense approach as is possible. There's the high protein, low carbohydrate diets. Then, there's the high carbohydrate, low protein diets. Not to mention the hundreds of other diets that tout the benefits of every kind of extreme dietary behavior possible. Stay away from these diets as if your health depended upon it. Because it does!

THE CAYCE APPROACH

Five elements combine to make up the well-rounded, balanced Cayce diet:

>An alkaline-producing diet
>Proper food combining
>Daily intake of grape juice
>A short list of diet "do's"
>A shorter list of diet "don'ts"

DIET

In a world where fad diets often test your mental abilities to plan and adhere to complicated dietary regimens, the Cayce diet is refreshingly simple and straightforward. It's based on a simple premise: Consume a diet that promotes a slightly alkaline condition in the body. The natural state of your body is a pH of 7.4, where 7 is neutral, more than 7 is alkaline, less than 7 acid. This chemical balance within the body is vital to good health.

Certain foods have a metabolic reaction within the body which produces an acid condition; others, an alkaline condition. By designing a diet that includes 80% alkaline-reacting foods to 20% acid-reacting foods, you can adequately balance your system for optimum health. Since the Cayce readings were innately health conscious, it is no surprise that this same diet tends to be low in fat and calorie content and high in fiber. Remember, these readings were given in the early part of this century, long before cholesterol became a household word.

THE "WEIGHT NO MORE DIET"

These are the basic guidelines for your daily diet:

Alklaine-Forming Foods
(80% of Your Diet)

All fruits except cranberries, plums, and prunes
All vegetables except for lentils and corn
All milk, including buttermilk
Almonds, brazil nuts, chestnuts, coconut, hazelnuts
Coffee, tea, molasses, brown sugar, brewer's yeast

Acid-Forming Foods
(20% of Your Diet)

All meats except for mincemeat
All cereals and bakery products except for soybeans
All cheeses and eggs
Peanuts, pecans, walnuts

TESTING YOUR ACID/ALKALINE BALANCE

One good way to test your acid/alkaline balance is by using blue litmus paper (found at most drugstores) to determine the pH of your saliva. The best time to take this test is in the morning before eating or drinking. Take a paper strip and wet it with your saliva. If the paper remains blue in color, the pH is alkaline at 7.0 or above. You're in safe territory.

If the strip turns pink, your saliva pH is below 7.0 or acid.

COMBINING TIPS

How you combine your foods is also critical to how they react within your body. The practice of eating the right foods together can have an immense impact upon the success of your diet. From the chart below try to combine in your daily diet the food category listed in the first column with that listed in the second column.

Food Type	Agrees	Disagrees
Starches	Vegetables	Milk, fruits, eggs, cheese, nuts, meats, sweets
Meats, seafood, fowl, nuts	Vegetables	Starches, milk, fruits, sweet desserts, cheese
Vegetables	All foods	
Dairy	Vegetables, fruits	Starches, meats, fish, fowl
Fruits (sweet)	Vegetables, dairy	Meats, fowl, seafood, eggs
Fruits (tart)	Vegetables	Starches, milk

THE GRAPE JUICE DIET

The grape juice diet is unique to the Cayce information. It was recommended in dozens of readings for people who needed to lose weight to improve their health and well-being. This diet is not one which works overnight; in fact, it requires persistency and consistency over a period of weeks and months. It is a routine which can be adopted for life to help your body reach its ideal weight and maintain it.

It works like this:

One-half hour before each meal and just prior to retiring at night, drink three ounces of Concord grape juice diluted with one ounce of water. Whenever possible, take five to ten minutes to sip the juice each time it is taken.

The Cayce readings indicate that many weight problems are the result of the body's assimilation processes being so out of whack that the cells and glands lining the walls of the intestines tend to extract and metabolize sugar from almost all foods. This can be one explanation why many people who eat the same quantities of food have dramatically varying weight patterns.

According to the readings, the grape juice helps balance the body's process of sugar metabolism. Interestingly enough, over 50% of the natural sugar in grape juice is fructose. Recent scientific studies have shown that a small dose of fructose prior to eating can decrease a person's appetite by roughly 30%. One can speculate that by satisfying the body's hunger for sugar just prior to food intake would help alter the abnormal behavior of these cells.

RUT TO RITUAL

As you begin to incorporate the grape juice into your diet, remember one thing: Don't make a chore of it. One item that threatens our busy lives is the deep sense of fulfillment we can derive from ritual. Rather than enjoying the life-sustaining activities we must undertake each day, we often allow those very activities to become dreary ruts of existence. We eat watching TV rather than enjoying each other's conversation. We take a drive to a neighbor's house rather than walk to it.

Begin to approach your day as a celebration of life. Slow down long enough to listen to the birds singing, to savor the aroma of fresh-cut grass. Stop and smell the roses. Does this advice sound cliche? Probably. But it is still powerful advice.

Build a ritual around your grape juice. Perhaps it becomes the five or ten minutes in the morning that you watch birds eating at the bird feeder. (If you don't have one, get one!) Use the time at midday to slow down before rushing through lunch. In the evening, sip the juice as you prepare a healthful evening meal. At night you might just wish to get cozy in bed with a good book and your juice.

If your responsibilities are such that it is unrealistic to expect such a surplus of quiet time, then work within your own personal demands. Perhaps you can find a way to create your ritual without feeling that you are neglecting your other responsibilities.

You get the idea. Don't dread having to remember the routine, just make it into a ritual that fits your style of enjoyment and look forward to it.

DIET DO'S

Seafood two or three times each week

Carrots, lettuce, and celery every day

Frequent vegetable and fruit salads prepared with gelatin

Lemonade (with no or very little sugar) as an afternoon drink

Grape juice, diluted with water, four times a day

Six to eight glasses of water a day

Honey as a sweetener

DIET DON'TS

No carbonated beverages

No potatoes (except the skins)

No fried foods

No white bread

Little cheese

Little pastry, cakes, and pies

MORNING, NOON, AND EVENING MEAL STRATEGIES

Mornings. Citrus fruits, followed with rice cakes or yoke of egg (not the white) poached, with a cereal drink, or black coffee or herbal tea. Or whole wheat or rye toast and egg yoke with cereal, coffee. Do not combine citrus with cereals or whole wheat at the same meal. Save your fruit for mid-morning.

Noons. Always a raw vegetable salad topped with a

moderate serving of salad dressing with an olive oil base. Use as many vegetables from above and below the ground as possible.

Evenings. Seafood, fowl, and occasional mutton. Soups. Above-the-ground vegetables.

Desserts? Yes! Occasional sherbet, fruit dessert prepared with gelatin, or fresh fruit sweetened with honey (from your local area if possible). All are on the menu. Enjoy them guilt-free!

EAT SLOWLY AND WITH A THANKFUL ATTITUDE

The Cayce readings indicated that bolting down food is a primary culprit in causing colds. Also, eating while upset or angry can have adverse effects on your health. In many ways, it's not simply what you eat that's important, but it's how you eat as well.

Thus, slow down and enjoy your meals. Cayce indicated that chewing foods thoroughly not only helps with digestion and assimilation but also helps keep the glands of the neck and face healthy.

As you eat, visualize the positive effects a healthy, balanced meal will have on your body and your energy level. Combine this with a thankful attitude, and you'll reap health-filled rewards.

EXERCISE

Without an increase in activity, any weight-loss program is destined to fail, either in the short or long run. Remember the bottom-line weight-loss formula: the calories you take in must be fewer than the calories you burn. If you simply cut calories, your metabolism will slow down to adjust for the shortfall in fuel, and your weight is likely to remain at a constant. Aerobic exercise is one of the only recognized ways that the body can and will adjust its "set point." The trick is to consume a comfortable, nutritious diet and increase your activity. Doing so will get the weight-loss formula working in the direction you desire.

For those who are inactive, the thought of exercise (especially aerobic) conjures up images of seemingly endless exertion and pain. Joggers running along the road grimacing with each stride. Basketball players glistening with sweat, hunched on the bench catching their breath. Or co-workers rushing off to an evening aerobics class. Fortunately, this is not the only form of exercise available to us. In fact, such extreme conditioning is and should be reserved for a small number of people who are and seek to be in exceptional shape.

WALKING IS YOUR BEST BET

Some form of aerobics should be the cornerstone of your exercise strategy. According to the Cayce readings, walking is the best of all exercises. If your walk is *brisk* enough to condition both heart and lungs, then you'll be gaining ground in your battle against excess pounds. It is a well-rounded activity, and if undertaken with the right attitude and spirit can be beneficial physically, mentally, and spiritually. When you plan and take your walks, remember these three items:

First, that you are walking both for enjoyment and to

get some aerobic conditioning. Set a pace that is slightly challenging, and stick with it. Choose a route you will enjoy and even consider timing your walks, so that you can *gradually* improve over a period of several weeks.

Second, enjoy the way your body feels as you walk. Be thankful that you have such a wonderful "friend" to carry you around. Stretch your muscles a bit as you walk, and feel the tension being released as you go along. Be happy!

Finally, decide if you like to walk alone or find a walking partner. Perhaps you'd like to listen to music or other cassette tapes that you've been meaning to listen to. Use this time in any way you want, especially if you're able to make it fruitful and fulfilling. As days go by and you consistently stay with your program, enjoy the feeling of accomplishment it gives you. Build on that feeling to increase your sense of self-esteem and self-confidence.

HEAD AND NECK EXERCISE

A specific, more general exercise for the head and neck was suggested in the Cayce readings over 300 times. It's very simple and has an almost immediate energizing effect. Here's how to do it.

Sit with your back straight and your shoulders relaxed. Take several deep breaths and let the tension fall away more and more with each exhalation. Now, slowly bend your head forward three times, backward three times, to the right three times, to the left three times. Then, gently rotate your head clockwise three times, counterclockwise three times.

Do this series slowly. A good time to do it is in the morning shortly after awakening, perhaps at noon if you have some time to relax, and in the evening before going to bed. Also, consider resting a moment on a bench or step while on your daily walk and practicing this therapeutic neck stretch. It should leave you relaxed and renewed.

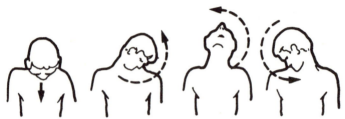

STRETCH LIKE A CAT

In general terms the readings recommended stretching like a cat as the ideal way to tone the body. If you can observe a cat, your own furry friend or a neighbor's, you'll find that cats are masters of their muscles. They are almost elastic in the way they stretch and can perform amazing feats from a standing-still position—for example, jumping four times their height and landing on a counter top without disturbing any of the items in their path (usually!).

Specifically, Cayce recommended that the upper body be exercised in the morning, the lower body in the evening. As you establish your own routine, keep this recommendation in mind. After all, it makes sense. In the morning, after you've rested, you need to pump up the blood to get ready for the demands of the day. At night, the opposite is true. You need to relax and draw the blood away from the head and neck, where tension is often stored, so that you can get a good night's rest.

MORNING STRETCH

A good morning exercise was described in Chapter Five in the discussion about increasing eliminations through the lungs. A simpler variation of that exercise is to stand straight and tall, then slowly rise up on your tiptoes, inhaling gently and deeply. Gradually bring your arms upward over your head. Then, still on your tiptoes, slowly bend forward and bring your fingertips down to touch your toes. Just as your hands near the floor, exhale forcefully in a single breath. Repeat three to ten times—whatever amount feels comfortable for you.

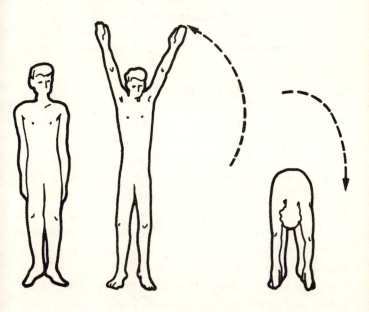

PELVIC ROLL

A specific evening exercise often recommended in the readings is the pelvic roll. Position yourself on your stomach as if preparing to do a pushup, but with your feet flush against the wall. Elevate yourself on your hands, then rotate your hips in a circle—three times clockwise, three times counterclockwise. Ideally, keep your elbows straight while you do this exercise. However, if it is too strenuous, you may actually rest on your elbows rather than your hands when you assume the pushup position.

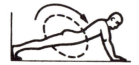 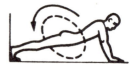

Circular motion

**clockwise
three times**

**counterclockwise
three times**

YOGA ANYONE?

Yoga, once a "far out" Eastern practice, is as at home in mainstream America today as Jane Fonda. Can this be true? Believe it or not, many of the exercise videos on the market today are full of basic yoga postures—not to mention the yoga videos that state up front what they are and how they can benefit your body, mind, and soul.

If you are the type of person who feels the need for a structured routine or exercise, consider purchasing a beginner's yoga video or even calling your local recreation center to see if a yoga class is on the schedule. Many public and cable television stations also feature yoga instruction programs. You may be pleasantly surprised that you're not the only person looking to the "ancients" for modern solutions to weight control and increased physical health and body flexibility!

A FINAL WORD ON EXERCISE

Use the above advice as a foundation for an exercise program with which you are comfortable. Remember that your goal is not to win an Olympic medal; it's to give your body a level of activity that promotes health and vigor. Combined with proper diet, exercise will be an effective tool in your weight-loss campaign.

Chapter Seven

THE FOUR-WEEK THERAPY PROGRAM

THE FOUR-WEEK THERAPY CYCLE

The following four-week therapy cycle provides you with a suggested routine to apply as you begin your new, healthful life style. You need to listen to your body (and your doctor or therapist) as you progress, making adjustments and changes as you feel are necessary.

Supplement this cycle with a healthy diet as recommended earlier, specifically observing its do's and don'ts. Of course, do regular exercises on a level that feels comfortable to you.

GETTING READY

- Set up an appointment with an osteopath or chiropractor who administers spinal adjustments and share with him or her your long-term goals. Listen to the feedback. Make sure that you are comfortable with the recommendations. Your relationship with your osteopath or chiropractor will be valuable and long-term. If you are uneasy about any aspect of your visit, get a second opinion. Your goal is to have a therapist whom you can trust.

- Follow the same procedure with a massage therapist and a colonic specialist. If you cannot find a professional who administers colonics, purchase the necessary supplies and equipment to give yourself a home enema. (See Appendix D.)

ROUTINE

Week One DAILY Keep up with your journal, work with your "Willpower Muscle Builders," and listen to your pre-sleep tape. (See Chapter Four.)

MONDAY Start "The Ideal You" exercise. Steam and massage.

MONDAY-FRIDAY Atomidine series.

TUESDAY Spinal adjustment.

TUESDAY-THURSDAY Castor oil packs.

FRIDAY Review and refine your "Ideal You." Colonic or enema.

FOUR TIMES A WEEK Fresh air and exercise.

Week Two DAILY Keep up with your journal, work with your "Willpower Muscle Builders," and listen to your pre-sleep tape. (See Chapter Four.)

MONDAY Review and refine your "Ideal You." Steam and massage.

TUESDAY Spinal adjustment.

TUESDAY-THURSDAY Castor oil packs.

THURSDAY Home steam or hot-tub routine.

FOUR TIMES A WEEK Fresh air and exercise.

Week Three DAILY Keep up with your journal, work with your "Willpower Muscle Builders," and listen to your pre-sleep tape. (See Chapter Four.)

MONDAY Review and refine your "Ideal You." Steam and massage.

TUESDAY Spinal adjustment.

TUESDAY-THURSDAY. Castor oil packs.

THURSDAY Home steam or hot-tub routine.

FOUR TIMES A WEEK Fresh air and exercise.

Week Four DAILY Keep up with your journal, work with your "Willpower Muscle Builders," and listen to your pre-sleep tape. (See Chapter Four.)

MONDAY Review and refine your "Ideal You." Steam and massage.

TUESDAY Spinal adjustment.

THURSDAY Home steam or hot-tub routine.

FOUR TIMES A WEEK Fresh air and exercise

EXERCISE: THE PLAN

The following Planning Worksheet will help you pull together your thoughts and plans for your new life style. Write out your answers in the spaces provided.

PLANNING WORKSHEET

1. There are good points about my body, and here's how I'm going to take better advantage of these physical assets:

2. I have positive qualities and abilities, and here's how I'm going to make better use of them:

3. I plan to drink my diluted grape juice _____ times daily during the following times:

To keep focused on how important this is, I may occasionally use a ritual like the following as I prepare to drink it:

4. I'm going to be sure to include these foods in my diet regularly:

5. I'm going to avoid these foods and these food combinations:

6. I will begin to walk _____ (frequency) for about _____ (how long) initially in the _____ (time of day). (For example: "I will begin to walk *three times a week* for about *½ hour* initially in the *mornings*.")

I am prepared to encounter the following obstacles to walking:

a) obstacles from inside myself:

b) obstacles from other people or conditions:

Here's what I plan to do to overcome these obstacles:

7. My main reasons and excuses for not having maintained my ideal weight in the past have been:

Recognizing this, here's what I can do to succeed:

8. I realize that I sabotage myself in trying to control my weight whenever I:

But instead I will now:

9. I recognize the following benefits or payoffs that I derive from staying at my current weight:

But, seeing this, I know that I can achieve the following goals which are more constructive if I achieve my weight-loss goals:

10. In the past, my well-intentioned efforts to lose weight didn't accomplish lasting results because of these competing demands and motives:

But now I plan to replace those demands and motives with these new ones:

11. I will take the time and energy it requires to be successful, without worrying that I am being selfish. For example, as an investment in myself and my goals, I will:

12. I can look at the difficulty controlling my weight as an opportunity for positive development and soul growth. I feel:

Conclusion

MEET THE NEW YOU

Once you begin this new program, what will your life be like? Will you feel miraculously better in a few days? Will you feel the same? Or worse? Beyond how you feel, when will the pounds start falling off?

Like many of the questions we raised throughout this book, there are no simple answers. There are certainly no promises. Every person is unique. We are each at a unique stage in our growth—physically, psychologically, and spiritually.

Some people may find that they actually gain weight for a few days when they start on a new diet. Some may lose five to seven pounds rapidly, and then level off. For the most part, this is a fluctuation in your body's water content. It can have a much more dramatic effect on your weight than the buildup and loss of body tissue, whether it be fat or muscle. Nevertheless, keep drinking six to eight glasses of water a day. This practice is vital to success.

What will happen over time is that you will begin to lose, slowly but surely. If you stick to a healthy life style and keep up with your grape-juice ritual, time will prove to be your greatest ally. You will feel better and look better—and your new "looks" will be much more than a slimmer, trimmer body. The "Weight No More Diet" will result in healthier, more radiant skin, clearer eyes, and—because you'll be succeeding—a brighter smile. Good luck!

APPENDIX A

WHO WAS EDGAR CAYCE?

Edgar Cayce exhibited unusual psychic ability at an early age and soon became known for his remarkable clairvoyant gifts. In a self-induced state, he was able to diagnose illnesses and prescribe remedies with remarkable success. Often referred to as "the sleeping prophet" and the world's most documented psychic, Edgar Cayce left behind a legacy of over 14,000 psychic readings covering such subjects as healing, dreams, meditation, reincarnation, prophecy, and psychic ability.

Born in 1877 in Hopkinsville, Kentucky, he discovered by accident that he could absorb information on any particular subject merely by napping for a while on a book pertaining to that topic. At the age of fifteen he suffered an accident, and, while in a coma, instructed his astonished parents to prepare a poultice to be applied at the base of his brain. The application fully restored him.

After he reached adulthood, his job as a salesman was threatened by a mysterious paralysis of the throat muscles which medical doctors were unable to treat. He consulted a hypnotist, and it was under the subsequent trance that Edgar correctly diagnosed his condition and prescribed an almost immediate cure.

Not long after, Edgar discovered that his gift could be used to help others, and what followed was over forty years of helping people from his self-induced state of unconsciousness. For 22 of these years, his readings were largely confined to medical problems; however, the scope of Edgar's abilities expanded in later years to include such subjects as meditation, dreams, reincarnation, and the Bible.

Edgar Cayce is regarded today as one of the most significant explorers of the human psyche in the twentieth century.

APPENDIX B

HOW THE A.R.E. CAN HELP YOU

A wealth of information from the Edgar Cayce readings is available to you on hundreds of topics, from astrology and arthritis to universal laws and world affairs, through the organization which Edgar Cayce founded in 1931, the Association for Research and Enlightenment, Inc.

The facilities and benefits offered by the A.R.E. include the largest body of documented psychic information anywhere in the world: the 14,263 Cayce readings, copies of which are housed in the A.R.E. Library/Conference Center in Virginia Beach, Virginia. These readings have been indexed under 10,000 different topics and are available to the public.

Membership in the A.R.E. is inexpensive and includes benefits such as: the bimonthly magazine, *Venture Inward;* home-study lessons in spiritual awareness and growth; the A.R.E. Library, available to you through book-borrowing by mail, offering collections of the actual Edgar Cayce readings as well as access to one of the world's best parapsychological book collections; and the names of doctors or health care professionals in your area who are willing to work with the remedies prescribed in the Edgar Cayce readings.

As an organization on the leading edge of exciting new fields of study, A.R.E. also presents seminars around the nation, led by prominent authorities in various fields and exploring such areas as parapsychology, dreams, meditation, personal growth, world religions, reincarnation and life after death, and holistic health.

The unique path to personal growth outlined in the Cayce readings is developed through a worldwide program of study groups. These informal groups meet weekly in private homes—right in your community—for friendly consciousness-expanding discussions.

A.R.E. maintains a visitors' center that offers a well-stocked bookstore, exhibits, classes, a movie, and audiovisual presentations to introduce seekers from all walks of life to the fascinating concepts found in the Cayce readings.

A.R.E. conducts ongoing research into the helpfulness of both the medical and nonmedical readings, often giving members the opportunity to participate in the studies themselves.

For more information and a free color brochure, write or phone:

A.R.E., P.O. Box 595
67th Street and Atlantic Avenue
Virginia Beach, VA 23451, (804) 428-3588

APPENDIX C

HOW TO OBTAIN A PRE-SLEEP TAPE FOR WEIGHT LOSS

The following pre-sleep tape is available to assist you in your weight-loss plan:

LOSE WEIGHT NATURALLY

The suggestions on this program will free you from the dead-end cycle of fighting your body and its desires. These positive suggestions will help you program your mind to:
- Control your appetite
- Create a slender self-image
- Control the stress caused by weight

Awaken a genuine love and respect for the body you want to create. Only then, according to Edgar Cayce, will you achieve results. **Cassette Tape 2106 $9.95**

This audiotape may be ordered from: A.R.E., 67th St. and Atlantic Ave., Virginia Beach, VA 23451; 1-800-368-2727.

APPENDIX D

DIRECTIONS FOR SELF-ADMINISTERED THERAPIES

Administering an Enema

Here are some basic guidelines for administering a home enema. First, gather the following items: enema bag, two large towels, Vaseline, plastic trash bag, alcohol, salt, pure spring water, Glyco-Thymoline, and sodium bicarbonate.

Begin by sterilizing the tube or nozzle of the enema bag with the alcohol. Prepare a quart of lukewarm spring water (body temperature), adding a teaspoon each of sodium bicarbonate and salt. Spread out a large plastic trash bag beneath several towels on the bed or floor and lie down on your left side. Have the bag elevated above the level of your body. Coat the enema nozzle with Vaseline and insert it two to four inches into your rectum. (Caution: Do not force it.) Allow one third of the water to enter your colon slowly. If you begin to cramp, clamp the tube closed and take several deep breaths. Then loosen the clamp and gradually continue. Once one-third of the water is inside, turn over on your back and allow the next third to enter, following the same procedure. Finally, shift to your right side and empty the remaining fluid from the bag into your body.

Now, try to hold the solution for five to fifteen minutes, moving gently to swish the fluid around the colon. This allows the fluid to soften and loosen the wastes. Your next step is to use the bathroom, where you can expel the water.

Rest a few moments, then repeat the process until the fluid which leaves your body is mostly clear. Administer a final enema, adding a teaspoonful of Glyco-Thymoline (which you can find at a health food store) to the water (instead of the salt and soda). This will serve as an antiseptic to the colon.

Setting Up a Home Steam

The first time you set up your home steam may seem involved, but once you have the routine down, it will be quite an easy process and one you will enjoy. You should attempt to find time for a steam about twice a month.

To set up a homemade steam cabinet, begin by gathering the following items: straight-backed wooden chair, old sheet, several towels, thermometer, hot plate, pie rack, pan of boiling water, custard cup, and oil or ingredient for steam additive.

Find a straight-backed chair, preferably wooden, which will not be damaged by short-term heat and moisture. Drape the back and legs of the chair in towels so that the rising steam or heated seat won't burn you. Make sure, however, that the steam can rise freely along the sides of the chair. Place a hot plate and pan of boiling water beneath the chair. Find an old sheet that you'll use as your "steam sheet" again and again. Cut a hole in the middle of the sheet, just large enough to fit your head through. Prior to your steam, drink three glasses of water. Now sit on the chair naked, draping the sheet around the chair like a tent. Be sure that the sheet does not come in contact with the hot plate. Wrap a towel around your neck to keep the steam from escaping.

For safety's sake, have a friend or family member near. This individual can provide you with drinking water which will keep your body fluids balanced and increase perspiration. Also, check your pulse periodically. It should stay below 140 beats per minute. Your temperature should remain below 104° F.

When your steam is finished, stand up slowly. Be sure you're not feeling faint, and proceed to the bathroom. Take a cleansing shower, then rub your body firmly with peanut oil, massaging your muscles and joints with deep, even strokes.

To aid in helping stimulate elimination, find a small glass or ceramic container (like a custard cup), and add a teaspoon of your choice of healing ingredient (one type only at any given steam). Float this cup on top of the boiling water or set it on the pie rack above the pan of water. The substance will vaporize as a result of the heat and help stimulate the skin. Common additives to use are: Atomidine, witch hazel, wintergreen, pine oil, tincture of myrrh, lavender oil, benzoin, and eucalyptus oil.

Applying a Castor Oil Pack

For preparing and applying a pack, gather these items:

Cold-pressed castor oil
2' square of wool flannel
Large towel
2 safety pins
Small plastic trash bag
Electric heating pad

Glass or ceramic bowl
Glass jar or plastic container

2 tsp. baking soda added to container with 1 quart of warm water

Pour heated castor oil into glass or ceramic bowl. Fold the flannel cloth four times to a 1' square. Place it in the bowl, saturating it with the oil. Wring out the excess. Now place the pack on the right side of your abdomen, positioned slightly toward the pelvic/liver area. Cover the pack with the plastic bag, put the heating pad on top of it, and place a towel on top of these layers, wrapping it around the body and fastening it with safety pins. Then turn on the heating pad. You may want to lie on a plastic bag or towel to protect the bedsheets.

A good routine is to apply the pack for one-hour periods in the evening three days in a row for three weeks. Leave off a week, and repeat the three-day/three-week cycle, using the same days of the week and times as before. (Women should not apply the pack during their menstrual cycle.) Store the pack in a glass jar or plastic container. Packs may be reused any number of times, but should not be used by another individual.

Dip a rag into the warm water with the baking soda and clean the abdomen. The oil will contain toxins brought out through the skin and, if the abdomen is not properly cleansed, these toxins will be reabsorbed.